Stretching Programs for Women's Health Issues

Womens Wellness Publishing, LLC
www.womenswellnesspublishing.com
www.facebook.com/wwpublishing

Mention of specific companies or products in this book does not suggest endorsement by the author or publisher. Internet addresses and telephone numbers for resources provided in this book were accurate at the time it went to press.

Cover design by Rebecca Rose

ISBN 978-1-939013-84-2

Note: The information in this book is meant to complement the advice and guidance of your physician, not replace it. It is very important that women who have medical problems be evaluated by a physician. If you are under the care of a physician, you should discuss any major changes in your regimen with him or her. Because this is a book and not a medical consultation, keep in mind that the information presented here may not apply in your particular case. In view of individual medical requirements, new research, and government regulations, it is the responsibility of the reader to validate health practices and treatments with a physician or health service.

Acknowledgements

I want to give a huge thanks to my amazing editors Kendra Chun and Sandra K. Friend for their incredibly helpful assistance with putting this book together. I also greatly appreciate my fantastic Creative Director, Rebecca Richards, as well as Letitia Truslow, my wonderful Director of Media Relations. I enjoyed working with all of them and found their help indispensable in creating this exceptional book for women. Most of all, I want to thank God and Jesus Christ for their love and blessings.

Table of Contents

Introduction

Dear Friend,

I have always loved doing stretching exercises. Even as a student in college and medical school, I was aware of how great stretching felt for my body. Stretches made me feel more vital, more alive and even more happy and joyful. I often combined stretching routines with the hiking and swimming that I loved to do on a regular basis. But it wasn't until I became a medical doctor with a busy practice treating thousands of patients that I began to explore the health benefits that specific stretches could have on helping to relieve many women's health issues.

Little children are naturally flexible, not only because their muscles and tissues are more supple and elastic but also because they are constantly moving around, stretching, playing, and jumping from place to place. As we get older, we become more immobile. Even as students we spend hours sitting in one position reading, writing papers, listening to lectures. As adults, many of us spend hours sitting at computers, doing deskwork, attending meetings or talking with clients. This lack of movement often aggravates health issues that we may already be suffering from since our muscles tend to shorten, contract and have impaired nutrient flow and lack of oxygenation to the affected parts of our body with immobility.

In this book, I share with you many wonderful stretching programs that I have developed over the years. In developing therapeutic programs for so many thousands of patients, I have looked at the research on exercise, including stretching and flexibility exercises, and have been very impr-essed by the benefits of physical fitness in creating health and wellness for my patients.

While I always counsel patients on the benefits of nutritional supplement-ation, a therapeutic diet, stress reduction and other therapeutic techniques; regular exercise and stretching programs can also bring relief to a wide variety of health issues. These have included arthritis, fibromyalgia, depression, anxiety, PMS, menopause, menstrual cramps, chronic fatigue, hypothyroidism, heart disease, high blood pressure and many other conditions.

Benefits of stretching exercises

Stretches are a wonderful antidote to our fast paced, over focused lives and provide effective relief from our daily stresses. I recommend that you perform them slowly and carefully and accompany the stretches with deep, relaxed breathing. Stretches quiet your mood and promote a deep sense of peace and calm. Unlike fast-paced aerobic exercise, stretches actually slow down your pulse, heart rate, and breathing. This benefits many women with anxiety and tension related to life stress. Stretches provide an oasis of calm in which you can put aside your daily stress.

When you practice a series of stretching exercises, you gently stretch every muscle in your body. This relaxes tense muscles and improves their suppleness and flexibility. These exercises also promote better circulation and oxygenation to tense and contracted areas throughout the body. As a result, general metabolism of the muscles and organ system is improved. Both the stress reduction effects and the physiological effects of stretching benefit all body systems, including digestive and elimination function, the endocrine (glandular) system, the nervous system, and the immune system. The brain, in particular, demands a healthy share of the body's available nutrients for optimal functioning. This is greatly benefited by practicing a regular stretching program.

Another way that stretching exercises help to reduce anxiety and calm the mood is by helping to balance the autonomic nervous system. The autonomic nervous system regulates the "fight or flight" response that many women experience with extreme stress. When this system is in overdrive, small life issues can become magnified out of proportion because the body reacts to these small stresses as if they were major life-threatening issues. Regular stretching and flexibility routines help to lessen the intensity of this response.

Gentle stretching and flexibility exercises also promote relief of pain and discomfort. When women are in pain, they tend to contract their muscles involuntarily. Tight and tense muscles in any part of the body have decreased blood flow and oxygenation. Waste products such as excessive carbon dioxide accumulate in this physical environment and can further worsen symptoms. In addition, pain causes breathing to become rapid and shallow. Less oxygen is taken in through respiration, which further decreases the oxygen available to the tight and tense parts of the body. Metabolism of the muscles becomes less efficient when this occurs.

Often, the areas where women have tight and tense muscles, ligaments, tendons and connective tissue correspond to the same areas of the body where they have health issues. For example, I have found that women with issues such as menstrual cramps, fibroid tumors and endometriosis often have tightness and tension of their pelvic muscles. Women with heart and lung disease often have tight and contracted muscles of the chest and upper back. Women with digestive complaints such as irritable bowel syndrome or indigestion may have tightness and tension in their upper or lower abdomen.

Stretching exercises can greatly help these underlying health issues by restoring elasticity and flexibility to the muscle in the affected parts of the body. In addition, they improve blood flow, oxygenation, nutrient flow and cellular energy to the affected organs and tissues which support the healing process. I consider them to be an essential part of any successful healing program. I hope that you enjoy these exercises, too!

If you are interested in exploring stretches for general fitness and flexibility and to improve and build your level of energy, I recommend my book, **Stretching and Flexibility for Women**.

Love,

Dr. Susan

1

Let's Get Started!

Motivating Yourself to Do a Stretching Program

If you encounter mental obstacles to beginning and sticking with a regular stretching program, there are many ways to overcome this resistance. It is helpful for you to pinpoint the exact cause of your resistance; this will make it easier to eliminate it.

- During the first week or two of your program, build up your exercise level gradually. Limit your initial stretching workouts to short sessions. For example, you might start out exercising every other day for only a few minutes. Then, increase the length of your sessions gradually in 5-minute increments until you are at the level that suits you the best.

- Perform the stretches in a relaxed and unhurried manner. Be sure to set aside adequate time so you do not feel rushed. Anytime you feel discomfort or excessive muscle tension, stop doing the exercise. Then re-evaluate your pace to see if it is too vigorous.

- Make sure you do your stretching program at the time of day that feels most natural. For example, if you are a late riser, don't try to exercise early in the morning. Exercise when you are the least hurried and stressed by your schedule. If your largest amount of free time is in the late afternoon between work and dinner, put aside that time to engage in physical activity.

- Do your stretches in an attractive setting. Some women enjoy stretching in a quiet area of their home while other women like to do their stretches outside in their yard or a park, weather permitting.

- You may want to do stretches with your partner, a friend or support person. This can be a great help in motivating and encouraging you to begin and stick with a stretching program.

- Use your mind to disconnect from your daily activities. Positive mental exercises can help you to relax before starting physical activity. Many women find that a few minutes of doing visualizations (seeing themselves performing and enjoying the stretching routine in their minds) or saying affirmations (positive statements about the benefits of exercise) can prepare them for a stretching routine.

- Listen to music while you do stretches. Many women find that the exercise period goes by much more quickly and the process is more fun and enjoyable when they listen to music. Be sure to choose music that is mellow and relaxing as it will help improve your mood and relax you further.

- Be sure to choose stretches that appeal to you and that you enjoy. Don't do stretches that worsen your stress level or that you find boring.

Beginning a Stretching Program

Before you begin your stretching program, read through the following guidelines; they will help you to perform your stretching program in an optimal manner and avoid any trauma or injury. These guidelines are particularly good for women who are just beginning a stretching program after leading a sedentary life. They are also helpful for women who have previously been fit and active but stopped exercising because physical exertion, including stretching, seemed to worsen fatigue or muscle tension.

- Only do stretches that seem to be appropriate for your level of health or fitness. A stretching program, or any other exercise routine, that is too strenuous can leave a woman feeling more tense, uptight or tired than ever.

- Do not do stretches that could promote injury to a part of your body that is already compromised.

- If you have any questions about the advisability of doing a particular stretching exercise or routine, then don't do those stretches. Choose stretches that, instead, seem to be appropriate for your level of health and fitness.

- If you have any questions about doing a particular set of stretches, I recommend that you check with your physician or health care provider to make sure that they approve before starting a program.

- Avoid doing stretches, or exercising, when you are ill or during times of extreme stress. At such times, the stress-reduction exercises or breathing exercises will be more useful.

- Move slowly and carefully when first starting to do a stretching program. This will help promote flexibility of the muscles and prevent injury. Follow the breathing instructions provided in the exercise. Most important, do not hold your breath. Allow your breath to flow in and out easily and effortlessly

- Always rest for a few minutes after finishing a session.

How to Perform Stretching Exercises

- I recommend that you try all of the exercises for your specific health issue during the first week or two of your program. However, if any of the exercises seem too difficult for your level of fitness, then it is best not to do those.

- The stretches should be performed in a relaxed and unhurried manner. Be sure to set aside adequate time—30 minutes or more—so that you do not feel rushed. Your exercise area should be quiet, peaceful, and uncluttered.

- Wear loose, comfortable clothing. It's better to exercise without socks to give your feet complete freedom of movement and to prevent slipping.

- Wait at least two hours after eating to exercise. Evacuate your bowels or bladder before you begin the exercises.

- Choose a flat area and work on a mat or a blanket. This will make you more comfortable while you do the exercises.

- Pay close attention to the initial instructions when beginning an exercise. Look at the placement of the body as shown in the photographs. This is very important, for you are much more likely to have relief from your symptoms if you practice the exercise properly.

- Try to visualize the exercise in your mind, then follow with proper placement of the body. This will help promote flexibility of the muscles and prevent injury. Follow the breathing instructions provided in the exercise. Most important, do not hold your breath. Allow your breath to flow in and out easily and effortlessly

- Move slowly through the exercise. This will help promote flexibility of the muscles and prevent injury. If you practice these stretches regularly in a slow, unhurried fashion, you will gradually loosen your muscles, ligaments, and joints. You may be surprised at how supple you can become over time.

- Always rest for a few minutes after doing the exercises. Try to practice these movements on a regular basis. A short session every day is best. If that is not possible, then try to practice them every other day.

2

Stretches for Relieving PMS

These stretches relieve specific symptoms of PMS including anxiety, depression, irritability, mood swings, and fatigue. They also help to relieve PMS related cramping, sugar craving, bloating, fluid retention, oily skin. These stretches energize the entire female tract as well as many internal organs. They help to relieve low back problems discomfort and stiffness, which can be aggravated with PMS, and bring blood flow and oxygenation to many internal organs.

Stretch 1

This exercise relieves low back pain and strengthens the spine. It improves blood circulation to the pelvic region and encourages chest expansion and lung elasticity. It also elevates mood and can help to relieve PMS related depression.

Lie on your stomach with your chin on the floor and your feet together. Place your palms flat on the floor, underneath your shoulders.

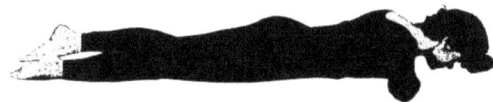

As you inhale, lift your head up, stretching your neck back. Then, raise your chest, using your arms and back muscles.

As you complete the inhalation, arch your body all the way up, keeping your hips on the ground.

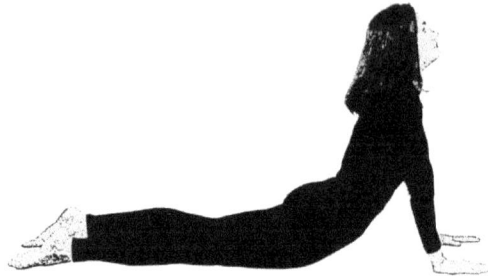

As you hold this position, exhale deeply. Then, breathe deeply and slowly, inhaling and exhaling for 30 seconds.

Lower yourself part way, using your arms for support. Holding the body at this angle, breathe deeply for 30 seconds.

Then let your body come all the way down. Relax with your head turned to one side and your arms resting gently on the floor. Close your eyes and relax for several minutes.

Stretch 2

This exercise strengthens the lower back, abdomen, buttocks, and legs. And prevents low back pain and cramps during the premenstrual period. It helps to reduce weight in the thighs and hips and tighten and firm the skin in these areas. It also energizes the entire female reproductive tract, thyroid, liver, intestines, and kidneys.

Lie face down on the floor. Make fists with both your hands and place them under your hips. This prevents compression of the lumbar spine while doing the exercise.

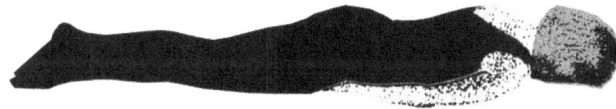

Straighten your body and raise your right leg with an upward thrust as high as you can, keeping your hips on your fists. Hold for 5 to 20 seconds if possible.

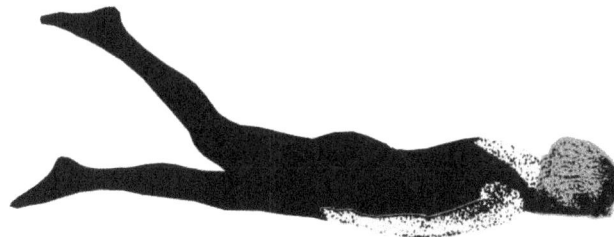

Lower the leg and slowly return to your original position. Repeat on the left side, then with both legs together. Repeat 10 times

Stretch 3

This exercise stretches the entire spine and helps to relieve low back pain and cramps. It stretches the abdominal muscles and strengthens the back, hips, and thighs. It also stimulates digestive organs and endocrine glands. It may help to relieve PMS related sugar craving, oily skin, and acne. And finally, it relieves PMS depression, fatigue, and lethargy, improving your energy and elevating your mood.

Lie face down on the floor, arms at your sides. Slowly bend your legs at the knees and bring your feet up toward your buttocks.

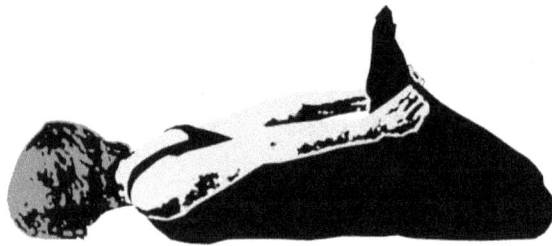

Reach back with your arms and carefully take hold of first one foot and then the other. Flex your feet to make grasping them easier.

Inhale and raise your trunk from the floor as far as possible. Lift your head and elevate your knees off the floor.

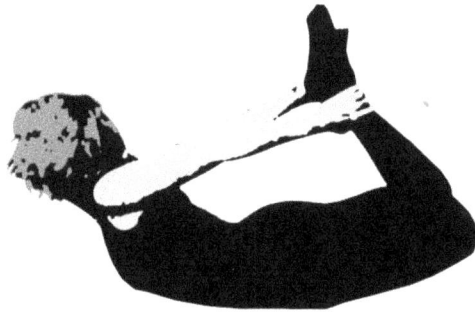

Squeeze the buttocks. Imagine your body looking like a gently curved bow. Hold for 10 to 15 seconds.

Slowly release the posture. Allow your chin to touch the floor and finally release your feet and return them slowly to the floor. Return to your original position. Repeat 5 times.

Stretch 4

This exercise gently stretches the lower back. It is excellent for calming PMS related anxiety and irritability. It also relieves menstrual cramps.

Sit on your heels. Bring your forehead to the floor, stretching the spine as far over your head as possible.

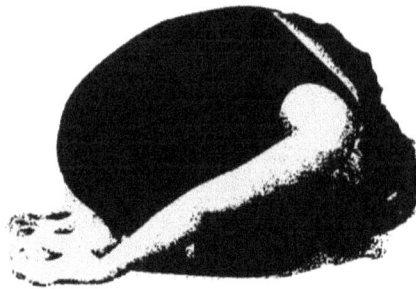

Close your eyes. Hold for as long as this is comfortable.

Stretch 5

This exercise opens the entire pelvic region, energizes the female reproductive tract, and relieves PMS related bloating and fluid retention in legs and feet.

Lie on your back with your legs against the wall and extended out in a V or an arc, and your arms extended to the sides.

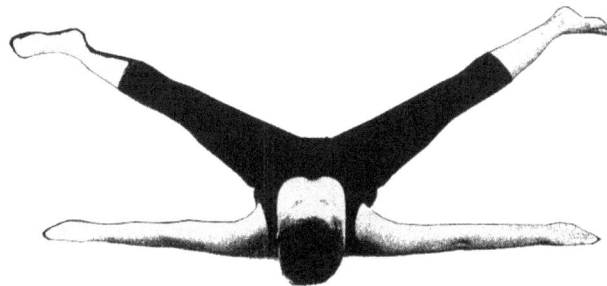

Hips should be as close to the wall as possible, buttocks on the floor. Spread legs apart as far as you can while still remaining comfortable.

Breathing easily, hold for 1 minute, allowing the inner thighs to relax.

Bring legs together and hold for 1 minute.

Stretch 6

This exercise improves the elasticity of the spine, strengthens the back and relaxes the abdomen and neck. It helps to reduce weight in the hips, thighs, legs, and abdomen. It improves circulation to the brain. It also reduces swelling and fluid retention in the legs and ankles.

Put a chair on your mat. Lie on your back, facing upward away from the chair. Arms are at your sides and palms are facing downward so that they press against the floor. Legs should be together.

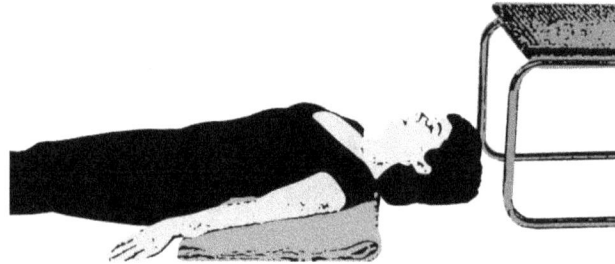

Slowly raise your legs and hips over your head until your toes touch the chair. This should be done without jerking, so bend your knees if necessary. Lift the spine by stretching the back muscles as much as possible. This exercise will alleviate compression of the lumbar spine.

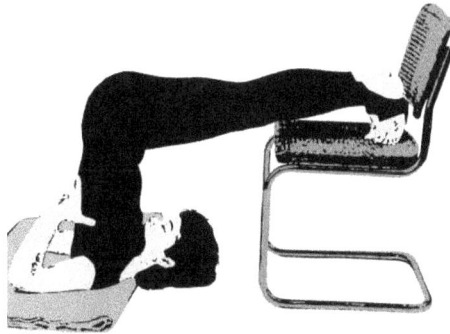

To come out of this posture, bend your knees and roll down slowly onto your back. Return to your original position.

(This exercise is usually done by bringing the legs and hips over the head until the toes touch the floor, but bringing the feet all the way to the floor could be harmful for women with PMS, since they often have a concavity of the back.)

Stretch 7

This exercise relieves anxiety and irritability and reduces eye tension and swelling of the face. It relieves menstrual cramps and low back pain if a rolled towel is placed under the knees.

Lie on your back with a rolled towel placed under your knees. Your arms should be at your sides, palms up.

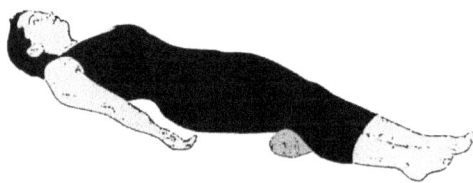

Close your eyes and relax your whole body. Inhale slowly, breathing from the diaphragm. As you inhale, visualize the energy in the air around you being drawn in through your entire body. Imagine that your body is porous and open like a sponge, so that this energy can be drawn in to revitalize every cell of your body.

Exhale slowly and deeply, allowing every ounce of tension to be drained from your body.

3

Stretches for Relief of Menstrual Cramps

Stretches can be tremendously beneficial in the treatment and prevention of menstrual cramps, pelvic congestion, and low back pain. The slow, controlled stretching movements that you do in these exercises help to relax tense muscles and improve their suppleness and flexibility. They also help to bring better blood circulation and oxygenation to the tense areas of your lower body, thereby improving the metabolism of the pelvic and back muscles. An additional benefit to stretches is that it helps to quiet your moods. The deep breathing and slow movement that accompany these exercises help to reduce anxiety and irritability and produce a sense of peace.

I have included a series of specific stretches poses that gently stretch every muscle in your body, with specific emphasis on the pelvic and low back region. As well as relieving cramps and discomfort, these exercises energize and balance the female reproductive tract and can help correct underlying hormonal imbalance through improved oxygenation and better circulation to the pelvic area. This can have a beneficial effect on menstrual function. Women who experience fatigue due to menstrual pain and discomfort can enjoy an increase in vigor and stamina when practicing the stretches exercises. I personally do stretches frequently as part of my own exercise routine.

Stretch 1

This exercise helps to relieve the low back tension that is so common with menstrual cramps. It also massages the neck and spine and flexes the vertebral column. It will invigorate and energize you, reducing fatigue. After doing this exercise, lie flat on your back for a few minutes to enhance the benefits of the exercise.

Lie on your back. Bend and raise your knees to your chest, clasping them with your hands. Hands should be interlocked below knees.

Raise your head toward your knees and gently rock back and forth on your curved spine.

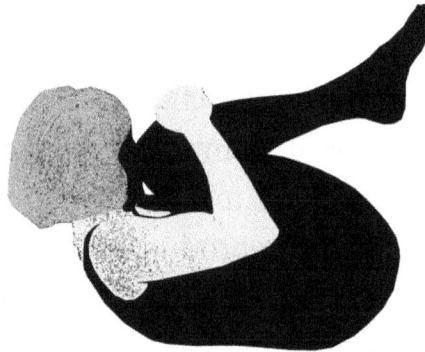

Note the roundness of your back and shoulders. Keep the chin tucked in as you roll back. Avoid rolling back too far on your neck. Rock back and forth 5 to 10 times.

Stretch 2

This is an excellent exercise for stretching the abdominal muscles which are often tightened with menstrual cramps. It is also helpful in reducing pelvic congestion.

Lie on your back with your knees bent. Spread your feet apart, flat on the floor.

Place your hands around your ankles, holding them firmly.

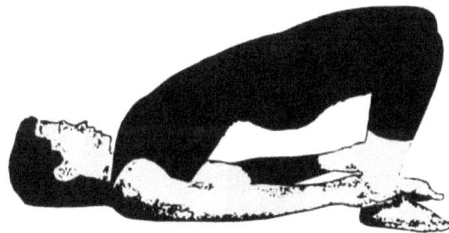

As you inhale, arch your pelvis up and hold for a few seconds. As you exhale, relax and lower your pelvis several times.

Repeat this exercise several times.

Stretch 3

This exercise flexes the low back, strengthening this area. By building this area up over time, you can help to prevent menstrual cramps and low back pain.

Kneel on all fours. As you inhale, arch your spine downward while your head goes back.

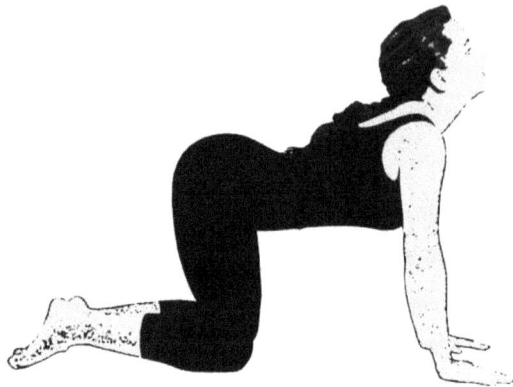

As you exhale, curve your spine into a rounded arch while your head goes down. Do this exercise in a rhythmic, fluid manner.

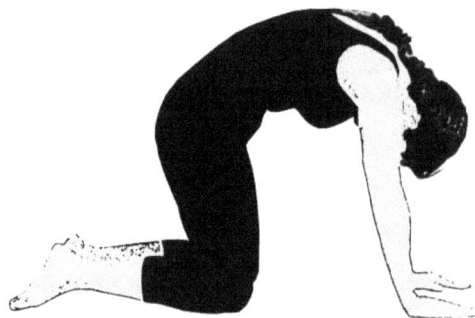

Stretch 4

This exercise strengthens the back and abdominal muscles. It also improves blood circulation and oxygenation to the pelvis, which helps to decrease cramps and calms anxiety and nervousness.

Lie down and press the small of your back into the floor. This permits you to use your abdominal muscles without straining your lower back.

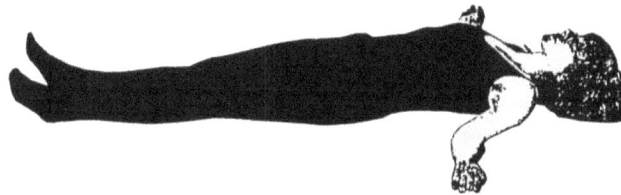

Raise your right leg slowly while breathing in. Keep your back flat on the floor and let the rest of your body remain relaxed. Move your leg up very slowly. Do not move your leg in a jerking manner. Hold for a few breaths.

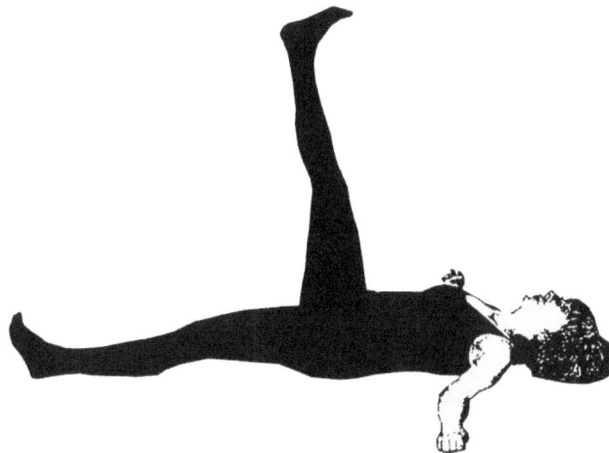

Lower your leg and breathe out. Repeat the same exercise on your left side. Then alternate legs, repeating the exercise 5 to 10 times.

Stretch 5

This exercise strengthens the lower back, abdomen, buttocks, and legs and helps to prevent low back pain and menstrual cramps. It also energizes the entire female reproductive tract. Regular practice of this exercise helps to improve posture and elimination. It helps to reduce weight in the thighs and hips and tighten and firm the skin in these areas.

Lie face down on the floor. Make fists with both your hands and place them under your hips. This prevents compression of the lumbar spine while doing the exercise.

Straighten your body and raise your right leg with an upward thrust as high as you can, keeping your hips on your fists. Hold for 5 to 20 seconds if possible.

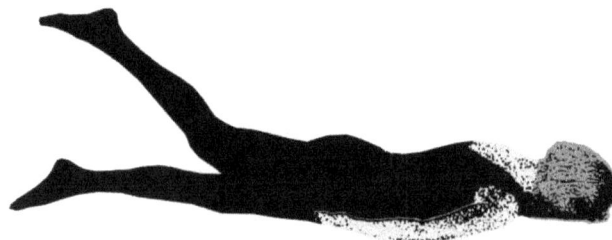

Lower the leg and slowly return to your original position. Repeat on the left side, then with both legs together. Repeat 10 times.

Stretch 6

This exercise stretches the entire spine and helps to relieve low back pain and menstrual cramps. It stretches the abdominal muscles and strengthens the back, hips, and thighs. It also stimulates the digestive organs and endocrine glands. Regular practice of this posture can help to relieve depression and fatigue, improving your energy and elevating your mood.

Lie face down on the floor, arms at your sides.

Slowly bend your legs at the knees and bring your feet up toward your buttocks.

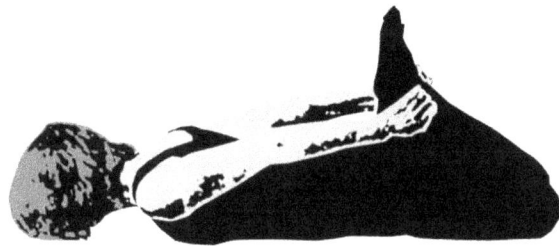

Reach back with your arms and carefully take hold of first one foot and then the other. Flex your feet to make grasping them easier.

Inhale and raise your trunk from the floor as far as possible. Lift your head and elevate your knees off the floor.

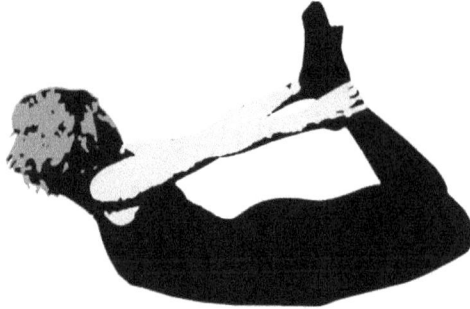

Squeeze the buttocks. Imagine your body looking like a gently curved bow. Hold for 10 to 15 seconds.

Slowly release the posture. Allow your chin to touch the floor and finally release your feet and return them slowly to the floor. Return to your original position. Repeat 5 times

Stretch 7

This exercise also gently stretches the lower back. It is excellent for calming anxiety and irritability. This is one of the most effective exercises for relieving menstrual cramps.

Sit on your heels. Bring your forehead to the floor, stretching the spine as far over your head as possible.

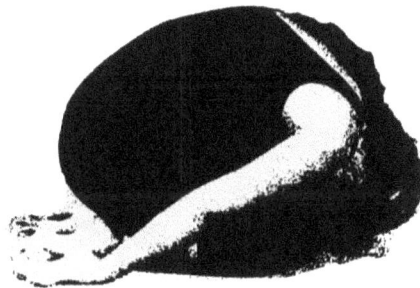

Close your eyes. Hold for as long as this is comfortable.

Stretch 8

This exercise helps to relieve the congestive symptoms that occur with menstrual cramps. It opens the entire pelvic region and energizes the female reproductive tract. It also relieves bloating and fluid retention in legs and feet.

Lie on your back with your legs against the wall and extended out like a V or an arc, and your arms extended to the sides.

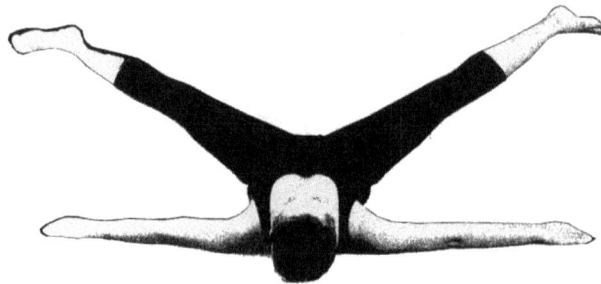

Hips should be as close to the wall as possible, buttocks on the floor. Legs should be spread apart as far as they can and still remain comfortable.

Breathing easily, hold for 1 minute, allowing the inner thighs to relax.

Stretch 9

This exercise relieves menstrual cramps and low back pain. It also relieves anxiety and irritability and reduces eye tension and swelling of the face.

Lie on your back with a rolled towel placed under your knees. Your arms should be at your sides, palms up.

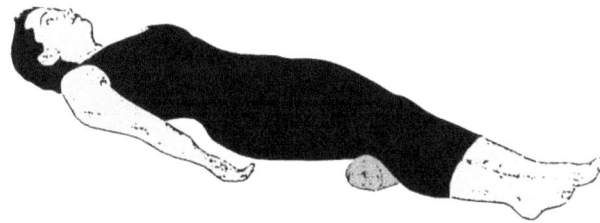

Close your eyes and relax your whole body. Inhale slowly, breathing from the diaphragm. As you inhale, visualize the energy in the air around you being drawn in through your entire body. Imagine that your body is porous and open like a sponge, so that this energy can be drawn in to revitalize every cell of your body.

Exhale slowly and deeply, allowing every ounce of tension to be drained from your body.

4

Stretches for Relief of Heavy and Irregular Menstruation

This chapter contains stretches that have a beneficial effect on menstrual function. The poses will also help reduce muscle tension in the pelvic area. For those women who are suffering from anemia due to heavy and irregular menstrual bleeding, these poses will provide the benefits of promoting oxygenation and better circulation to the pelvic area These stretches will gently move and lengthen many muscles in your body and will energize and balance the female reproductive tract.

Stretch 1

This exercise improves blood circulation through the pelvis and thereby stabilizes menstrual function. It helps to calm anxiety and also strengthens the back and abdominal muscles.

Lie down and press the small of your back into the floor. This permits you to use your abdominal muscles without straining your lower back.

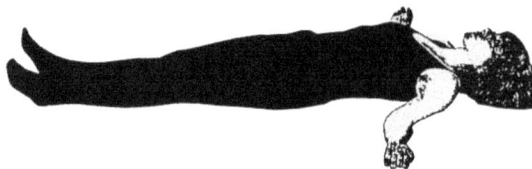

Raise your right leg slowly while breathing in. Keep your back flat on the floor and remain relaxed. Move your leg very slowly and smoothly.

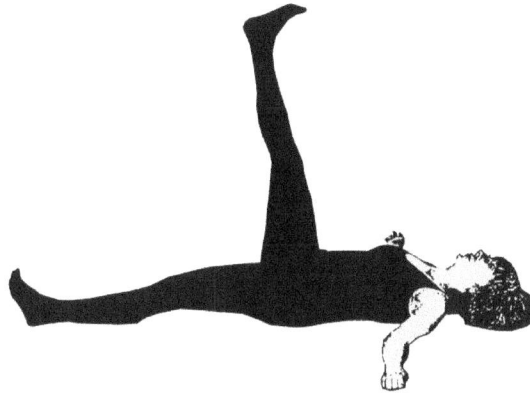

Hold for a few breaths. Lower your leg and breathe out.

Repeat the same exercise with your left leg. Then alternate legs, repeating 5 to 10 times.

Stretch 2

This exercise energizes and rejuvenates the female reproductive tract and tones the abdominal organs (pancreas, liver, and adrenals). It emphasizes freer pelvic movement with controlled breathing.

Lie on your back with your knees bent and your feet on the floor close to your buttocks.

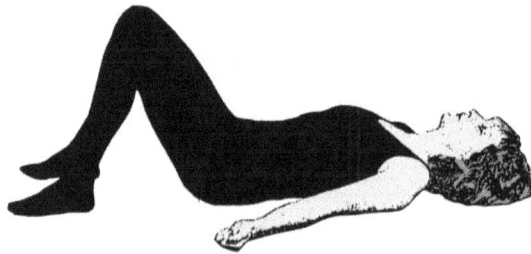

Exhale and press the lower back into the floor, raising the buttocks slightly. Arch the back slightly.

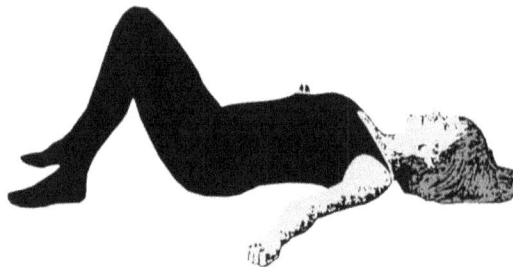

Inhale and lift your lower back off the floor. This stretches the region from the sternum to the pelvis.

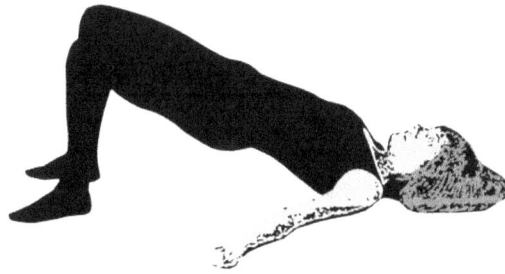

Repeat this exercise 10 times. Always lift your navel up on the in-breath. Always elongate your spine and press the lower back down on the out-breath.

Stretch 3

This exercise energizes the entire female reproductive tract, thyroid, liver, intestines, and kidneys. It may be helpful for women with anemia due to dysfunctional bleeding by improving circulation and oxygenation to the pelvic region. This exercise also strengthens the lower back, abdomen, buttocks, and legs, and prevents lower back pain and cramps.

Lie face down on the floor. Make fists with both your hands and place them under your hips. This prevents compression of the lumbar spine while doing the exercise.

Straighten your body and raise your right leg with an upward thrust as high as you can, keeping your hips on your fists. Hold for 5 to 20 seconds if possible.

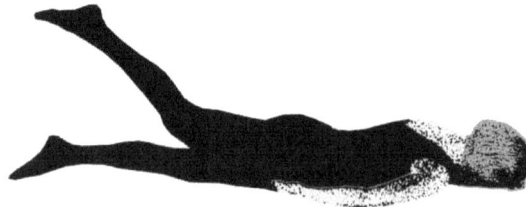

Lower the leg and slowly return to your original position. Repeat with the left leg, then with both legs together. Repeat 10 times.

Stretch 4

This exercise helps to relieve anemia-related fatigue and lack of vitality due to heavy and irregular menstruation, elevating your mood and improving stamina. This exercise also stretches the entire spine and helps to relieve lower back pain and cramps. It stretches the abdominal muscles and strengthens the back, hips, and thighs. It also stimulates the digestive organs and endocrine glands.

Lie face down on the floor, arms at your sides.

Slowly bend your legs at the knees and bring your feet up toward your buttocks.

Reach back with your arms and carefully take hold of first one foot and then the other. Flex your feet to make grasping them easier.

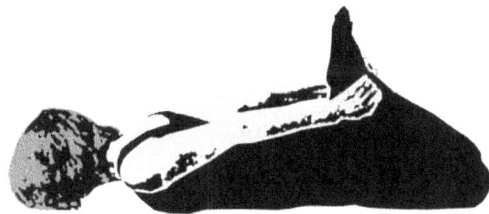

Inhale and raise your trunk from the floor as far as possible and lift your head. Bring your knees as close together as possible.

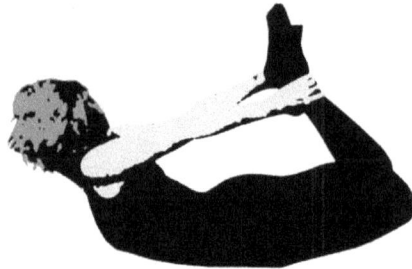

Squeeze the buttocks while raising them off the floor. Imagine your body looking like a gently curved bow. Hold for 10 to 15 seconds.

Slowly release the posture. Allow your chin to touch the floor and finally release your feet and return them slowly to the floor. Return to your original position. Repeat 5 times.

Stretch 5

This exercise opens the entire pelvic region and energizes the female reproductive tract. It is helpful for varicose veins and improves circulation in the legs.

Lie on your back with your legs against the wall and extended out in a V or an arc, and your arms extended to the sides.

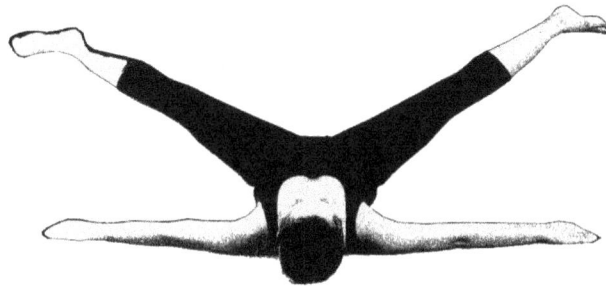

Hips should be as close to the wall as possible, buttocks on the floor. Spread legs apart as far as you can while still remaining comfortable.

Breathing easily, hold for 1 minute, allowing the inner thighs to relax. Bring legs together and hold for 1 minute.

5

Stretches for Relief of Endometriosis

The uncomfortable symptoms of endometriosis respond well to gentle stretches. Stretching exercises that emphasize pelvic movement and flexibility can help treat the menstrual cramps, pelvic congestion, and low back pain that commonly occur with this problem. Stretches may even help control heavy menstrual flow.

The slow, controlled stretching movements that you do in these exercises help relax tense muscles and improve their suppleness and flexibility. They also bring better blood circulation and oxygenation to the tense areas of your lower body, thereby improving the metabolism of the pelvic and back muscles.

Stretches have an additional benefit in that it quiets your moods. The deep breathing and slow movements that characterize these exercises reduce anxiety and irritability and produce a sense of peace—a welcome change for women who have endometriosis and also have significant life stress. The stress reduction effects of stretches benefit all body systems, including the reproductive tract and the immune system.

Stretch 1

This exercise helps stretch and release the low back and pelvic area. Besides relaxing this area and relieving pain, it also helps relieve hemorrhoids and constipation.

Sit on the floor with your legs placed straight out in front of you. Bend your right knee and place your right heel in your crotch area. Your left leg remains in a straight position.

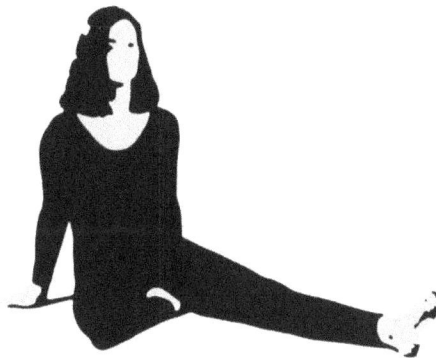

As you inhale, take hold of your left ankle, straightening your spine. Hold this position for 30 seconds.

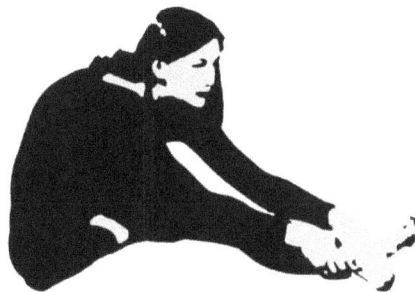

As you exhale, bring your forehead toward your left knee. Hold this position for 30 seconds. Repeat this exercise with the other leg.

Stretch 2

This is an excellent exercise for stretching the abdominal muscles that are often tightened with menstrual cramps and pain caused by endometriosis. It is also helpful in reducing the pelvic congestion that occurs when PMS coexists with these conditions.

Lie on your back with your knees bent. Spread your feet apart, flat on the floor.

Place your hands around your ankles, holding them firmly.

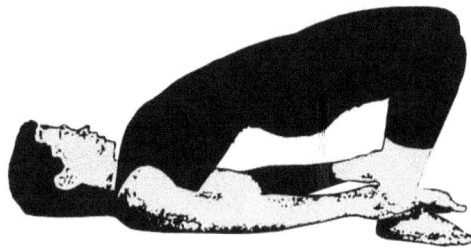

As you inhale, arch your pelvis up and hold for a few seconds. As you exhale, relax and lower your pelvis.

Repeat this exercise several times.

Stretch 3

This exercise strengthens the lower back, abdomen, buttocks, and legs, and relieves low back pain and menstrual cramps related to endometriosis. It also energizes the entire female reproductive tract. Regular practice of this exercise helps improve posture and elimination and will tighten and firm the thighs and hips.

Lie face down on the floor. Make fists with both your hands and place them under your hips. This prevents compression of the lumbar spine while doing the exercise.

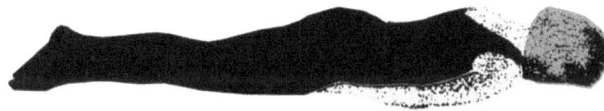

Straighten your body and raise your right leg with a slow upward thrust as high as you can, keeping your hips on your fists. Hold for 5 to 20 seconds if possible.

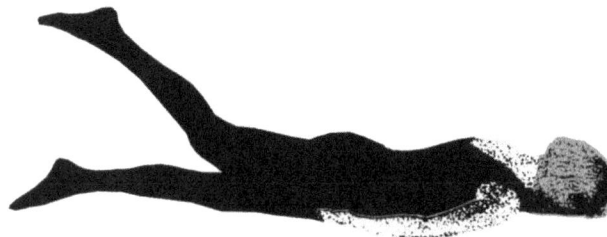

Lower the leg and slowly return to your original position. Repeat with the left leg, then with both legs together. Repeat 10 times.

Stretch 4

This exercise stretches the entire spine and helps relieve low back pain and menstrual cramps due to endometriosis. It stretches the abdominal muscles and strengthens the back, hips, and thighs. It also stimulates the digestive organs and endocrine glands. Regular practice of this posture can relieve depression and fatigue by improving your energy and elevating your mood.

Lie face down on the floor, arms at your sides. Slowly bend your legs at the knees and bring your feet up toward your buttocks.

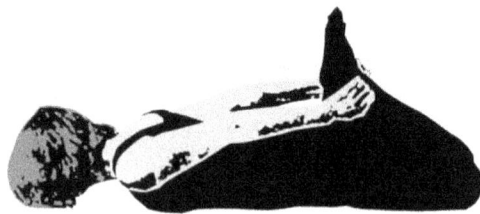

Reach back with your arms and carefully take hold of first one foot and then the other. Flex your feet to make grasping them easier.

Inhale and raise your trunk from the floor as far as possible. Lift your head and elevate your knees off the floor.

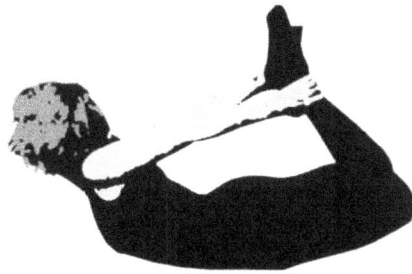

Squeeze the buttocks. Imagine your body looking like a gently curved bow. Hold for 10 to 15 seconds.

Slowly release the posture. Allow your chin to touch the floor and finally release your feet and return them slowly to the floor. Return to your original position. Repeat 5 times.

Stretch 5

This exercise gently stretches the lower back. It is excellent for calming anxiety and irritability. Many of my patients with menstrual cramps related to endometriosis practice this exercise often.

Sit on your heels. Bring your forehead to the floor, stretching the spine as far over your head as possible.

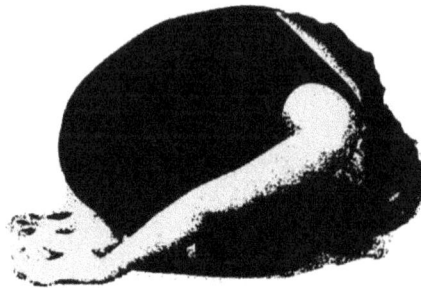

Close your eyes. Hold for as long as comfortable.

Stretch 6

This is another excellent exercise for endometriosis related pain and cramps. It is also useful for reducing symptoms in women with coexisting PMS and helps to relieve the congestive symptoms that occur with menstrual cramps. This stretch opens the entire pelvic region and energizes the female reproductive tract; it also relieves bloating and fluid retention in legs and feet.

Lie on your back with your legs against the wall and extended out in a V or an arc, and your arms extended to the sides.

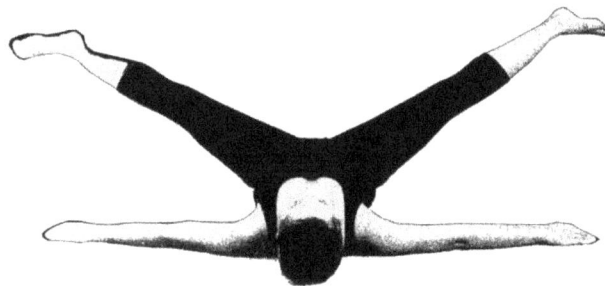

Hips should be as close to the wall as possible, buttocks on the floor. Spread legs apart as far as you can while still remaining comfortable.

Breathing easily, hold for 1 minute, allowing the inner thighs to relax.

6

Stretches for Relief of Fibroids

The uncomfortable symptoms of fibroids respond well to gentle stretches. Stretching exercises that emphasize pelvic movement and flexibility can help treat the menstrual cramps, pelvic congestion, and low back pain that commonly occur with this problem. Stretches may even help control heavy menstrual flow. The slow, controlled stretching movements that you do in these exercises help relax tense muscles and improve their suppleness and flexibility. They also bring better blood circulation and oxygenation to the tense areas of your lower body, thereby improving the metabolism of the pelvic and back muscles.

Stretches have an additional benefit in that it quiets your moods. The deep breathing and slow movements that characterize these exercises reduce anxiety and irritability and produce a sense of peace — a welcome change for women who have fibroids and also have significant life stress. The stress reduction effects of stretches benefit all body systems, including the reproductive tract and the immune system.

Stretch 1

This exercise helps stretch and release the low back and pelvic area. Besides relaxing this area and relieving pain, it also helps relieve hemorrhoids and constipation due to fibroid tumors.

Sit on the floor with your legs placed straight out in front of you. Bend your right knee and place your right heel in your crotch area. Your left leg remains in a straight position.

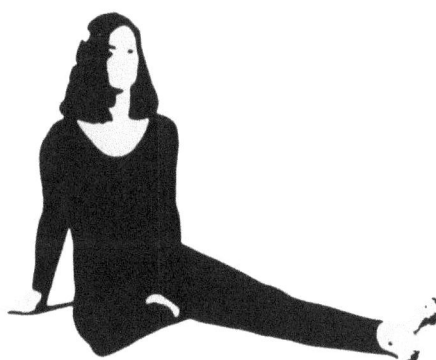

As you inhale, take hold of your left ankle, straightening your spine. Hold this position for 30 seconds.

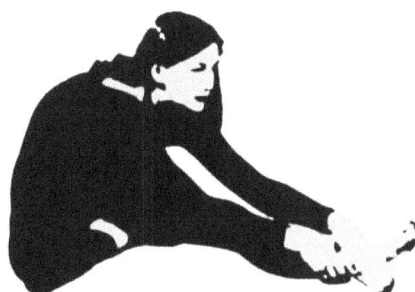

As you exhale, bring your forehead toward your left knee. Hold this position for 30 seconds. Repeat this exercise with the other leg.

Stretch 2

This is an excellent exercise for stretching the abdominal muscles that are often tightened with menstrual cramps and pain caused by fibroid tumors. It is also helpful in reducing the pelvic congestion that occurs when PMS coexists with these conditions.

Lie on your back with your knees bent. Spread your feet apart, flat on the floor.

Place your hands around your ankles, holding them firmly.

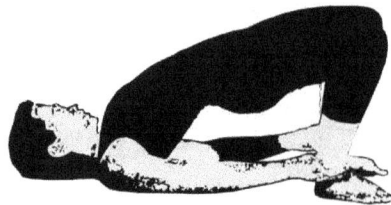

As you inhale, arch your pelvis up and hold for a few seconds. As you exhale, relax and lower your pelvis.

Repeat this exercise several times.

Stretch 3

This exercise strengthens the lower back, abdomen, buttocks, and legs, and relieves low back pain and menstrual cramps due to fibroids. It also energizes the entire female reproductive tract. Regular practice of this exercise helps improve posture and elimination and will tighten and firm the thighs and hips.

Lie face down on the floor. Make fists with both your hands and place them under your hips. This prevents compression of the lumbar spine while doing the exercise.

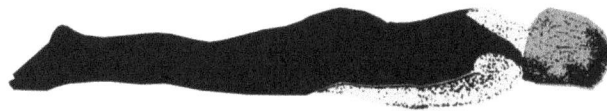

Straighten your body and raise your right leg with a slow upward thrust as high as you can, keeping your hips on your fists. Hold for 5 to 20 seconds if possible.

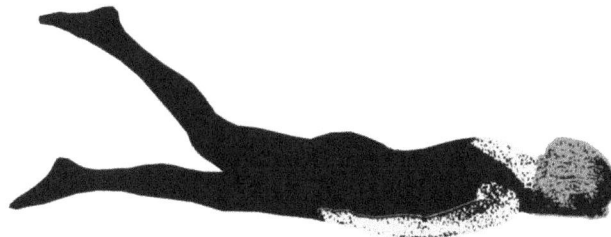

Lower the leg and slowly return to your original position. Repeat with the left leg, then with both legs together. Remember to keep your hips resting on your fists. Repeat 10 times.

Stretch 4

This exercise stretches the entire spine and helps relieve low back pain and menstrual cramps due to fibroids. It stretches the abdominal muscles and strengthens the back, hips, and thighs. It also stimulates the digestive organs and endocrine glands. Regular practice of this posture can relieve depression and fatigue by improving your energy and elevating your mood.

Lie face down on the floor, arms at your sides.

Slowly bend your legs at the knees and bring your feet up toward your buttocks.

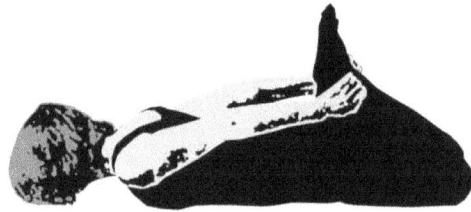

Reach back with your arms and carefully take hold of first one foot and then the other. Flex your feet to make grasping them easier.

Inhale and raise your trunk from the floor as far as possible. Lift your head and elevate your knees off the floor.

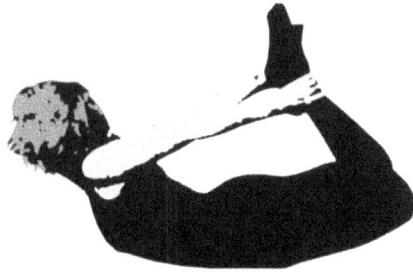

Squeeze the buttocks. Imagine your body looking like a gently curved bow. Hold for 10 to 15 seconds.

Slowly release the posture. Allow your chin to touch the floor and finally release your feet and return them slowly to the floor. Return to your original position. Repeat 5 times.

Stretch 5

This exercise gently stretches the lower back. It is excellent for calming anxiety and irritability. Many of my patients with menstrual cramps practice this exercise often.

Sit on your heels. Bring your forehead to the floor, stretching the spine as far over your head as possible.

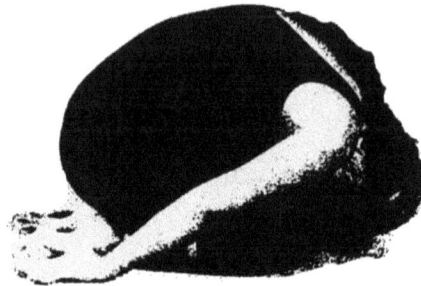

Close your eyes. Hold for as long as comfortable.

Stretch 6

This is another excellent exercise for menstrual related pain and cramps due to fibroids. It is also useful for reducing symptoms in women with coexisting PMS and helps to relieve the congestive symptoms that occur with menstrual cramps. This stretch opens the entire pelvic region and energizes the female reproductive tract; it also relieves bloating and fluid retention in legs and feet.

Lie on your back with your legs against the wall and extended out in a V or an arc, and your arms extended to the sides.

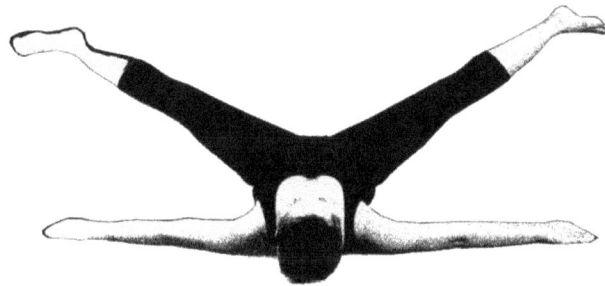

Hips should be as close to the wall as possible, buttocks on the floor. Spread legs apart as far as you can while still remaining comfortable.

Breathing easily, hold for 1 minute, allowing the inner thighs to relax.

7

Stretches for Relief of Menopause Symptoms

In this chapter, I present a series of stretches that promote more suppleness and flexibility to the entire body. This is very important for women in menopause since the muscles, ligament and tendons and their underlying connective tissues tends to tighten, shrink and contract with the decreased production of female hormones. The stretches also support the health of the ovaries, uterus and vagina because of the increased circulation and oxygenation to the pelvic area. Finally, practicing these stretches on a regular basis helps to balance the mood as well as support nervous system and brain function, which is very important during this time of life.

Stretch 1

This exercise energizes the entire female reproductive tract, thyroid, liver, intestines and kidneys. It is helpful for premenopausal women with dysfunctional bleeding, as well as women with menopausal symptoms such as hot flashes, because it improves circulation and oxygenation to the pelvic region, thereby promoting healthier ovarian function. This exercise also strengthens the lower back, abdomen, buttocks, and legs, and prevents lower back pain and cramps.

Lie face down on the floor. Make fists with both your hands and place them under your hips. This prevents compression of the lumbar spine while doing the exercise.

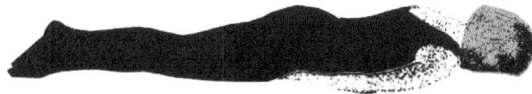

Straighten your body and raise your right leg with an upward thrust as high as you can, keeping your hips on your fists. Hold for 5 to 20 seconds if possible.

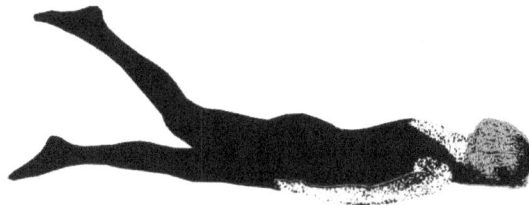

Lower the leg and slowly return to your original position. Repeat on the left side, then with both legs together. Repeat 10 times.

Stretch 2

This exercise improves blood circulation through the pelvis, thereby promoting healthier ovarian function. It helps relieve menopausal symptoms such as hot flashes and controls excessive bleeding in premenopausal women. The exercise helps calm anxiety and also strengthens the back and abdominal muscles.

Lie down and press the small of your back into the floor. This permits you to use your abdominal muscles without straining your lower back.

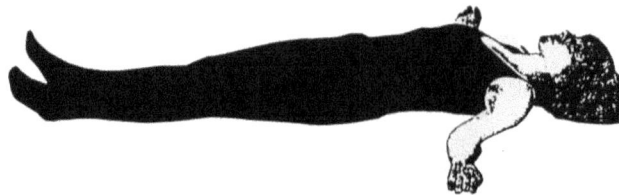

Keep your back flat on the floor and let the rest of your body remain relaxed.

Raise your right leg slowly while breathing in. Move your leg very slowly; imagine your leg being pulled up smoothly by a spring. Do not move your leg in a jerking manner. Hold for a few breaths.

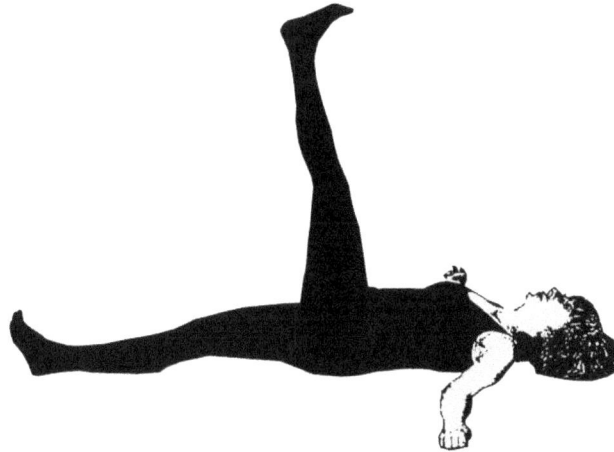

Lower your leg and breathe out. Repeat the same exercise on your left side. Then alternate legs, repeating the exercise 5 to 10 times.

Stretch 3

This exercise opens the entire pelvic region and energizes the female reproductive tract, improving ovarian function as well as normalizing excessive or irregular menstrual flow; diminution of menopausal symptoms may also occur. It is helpful for varicose veins and improves circulation in the legs.

Lie on your back with your legs against the wall and extended out in a V or an arc, and your arms extended to the sides.

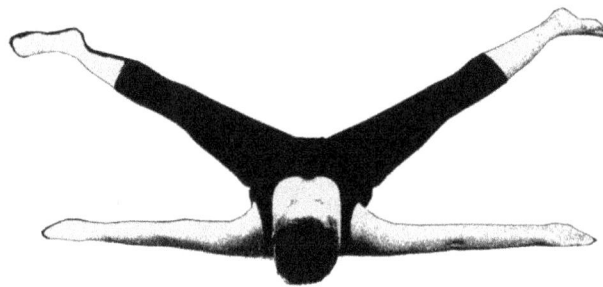

Hips should be as close to the wall as possible, buttocks on the floor. Spread legs apart as far as you can while still remaining comfortable.

Breathing easily, hold for 1 minute, allowing the inner thighs to relax.

Stretch 4

This exercise energizes and rejuvenates the female reproductive tract and tones the abdominal organs (pancreas, liver and adrenals). It emphasizes freer pelvic movement with controlled breathing.

Lie on your back with your knees bent and your feet on the floor close to your buttocks.

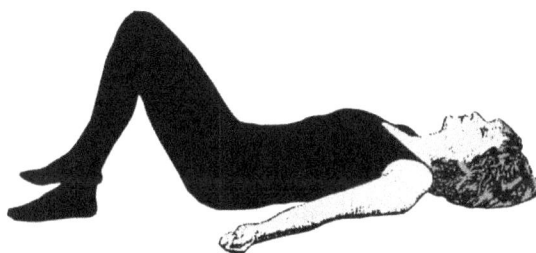

Exhale and press the lower back into the floor, raising the buttocks slightly. Arch the back slightly.

Inhale and lift your lower back off the floor. This stretches the region from the sternum to the pelvis.

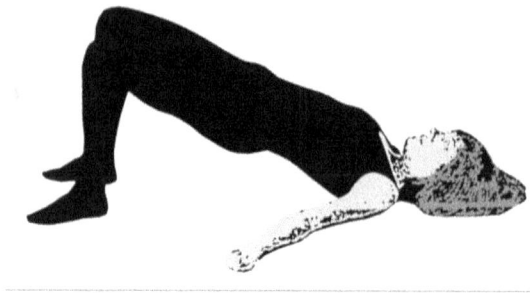

Repeat this exercise 10 times. Always lift your navel up on the in-breath. Always elongate your spine and press the lower back down on the out-breath.

Stretch 5

This exercise helps relieve menopause-related fatigue and lack of vitality, elevating your mood and improving stamina. The exercise also stretches the entire spine and helps relieve lower back pain and cramps. It stretches the abdominal muscles and strengthens the back, hips and thighs. It also stimulates the digestive organs and endocrine glands.

Lie face down on the floor, arms at your sides.

Slowly bend your legs at the knees and bring your feet up toward your buttocks.

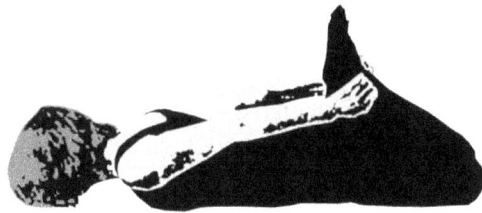

Reach back with your arms and carefully take hold of first one foot and then the other. Flex your feet to make grasping them easier.

Inhale and raise your trunk from the floor as far as possible. Lift your head and elevate your knees off the floor.

Squeeze the buttocks. Imagine your body looking like a gently curved bow. Hold for 10 to 15 seconds.

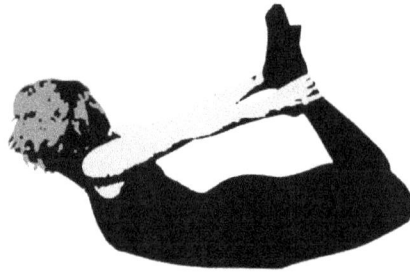

Slowly release the posture. Allow your chin to touch the floor and finally release your feet and return them slowly to the floor. Return to your original position. Repeat 5 times.

Stretch 6

This exercise is excellent for calming anxiety and stress due to emotional causes. This exercise will also relieve menopause-related anxiety and irritability. It gently stretches the lower back and is one of the most effective exercises for relieving menstrual cramps and low back pain.

Sit on your heels. Bring your forehead to the floor, stretching the spine as far over your head as possible.

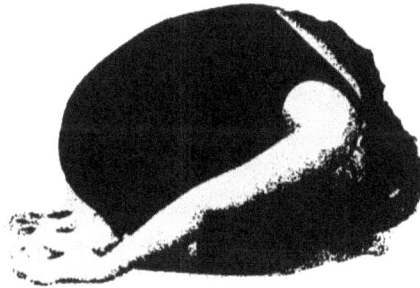

Close your eyes. Hold for as long as this is comfortable.

Stretch 7

This exercise relieves anxiety and stress due to emotional causes or menopause-related anxiety and tension. It relieves menstrual cramps and low back pain as well as reducing eye tension and swelling in the face.

Lie on your back with a rolled towel placed under your knees. Your arms should be at your sides, palms up.

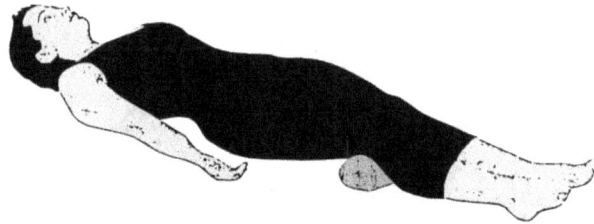

Close your eyes and relax your whole body. Inhale slowly, breathing from the diaphragm. As you inhale, visualize the energy in the air around you being drawn in through your entire body. Imagine that your body is porous and open like a sponge, so that this energy can be drawn in to revitalize every cell of your body.

Exhale slowly and deeply, allowing every ounce of tension to be drained from your body.

Stretch 8

This pose reduces anxiety and nervous tension and will help eliminate tension headaches and insomnia. It improves flexibility of the spine, reducing stiffness and back pain.

Lie on your back with your legs bent and your feet together. Place your hands on the sides of both ankles to keep your legs together.

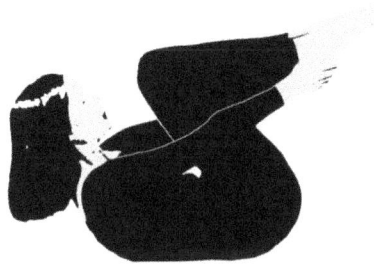

As you inhale, raise your legs up over your head. Make sure that the posture is comfortable by adjusting the angle of your legs. To do this, bend your knees to apply pressure between the shoulder blades.

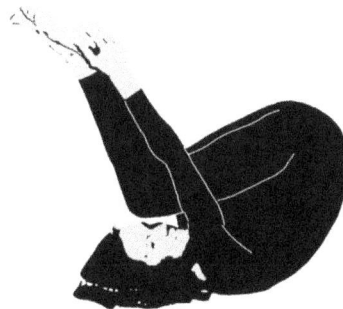

Hold this posture for one minute, breathing slowly and deeply. Return to the original position, lying flat on your back with your eyes closed. Relax in this position for several minutes.

Stretch 9

If your goal is to strengthen bone mass by increasing weight bearing on the legs, hips and spine, this exercise will help you accomplish increasing bone mass. It also improves balance and posture.

Standing straight, focus your eyes on a stationary point. Place one foot against the opposite thigh, so that one leg is bearing your weight.

Slowly raise your arms over your head. Hold for a count of 5. Reverse sides. Repeat 3 times.

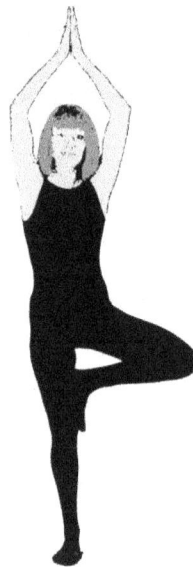

Note: You may place one hand on the wall for support if needed.

Stretch 10

This exercise increases circulation to the upper half of the body, energizing and stimulating the body. It also loosens and stretches tense muscles in the upper body, especially the shoulder and back, and expands the lungs.

Stand easily. Arms should be at your sides; feet are hip distance apart.

Bring your arms back slowly and gracefully until you can clasp them behind your back.

Exhale, then straighten your clasped hands and arms as far as you can without discomfort. Remember to stand upright; body should not bend forward. Breathe deeply into chest.

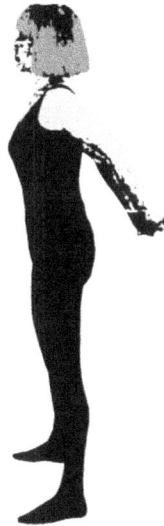

As you hold your breath, bend forward at the waist, bringing your clasped hands and arms up over your back. Relax your neck muscles and keep your knees straight. Hold for a few seconds.

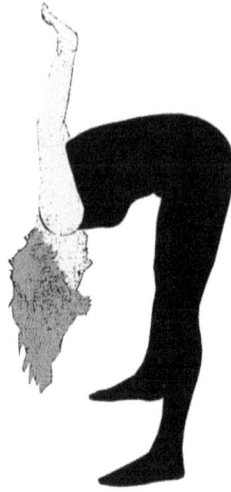

Exhale as you return to the upright position. Unclasp your hands and allow your arms to rest easily at your sides. Repeat sequence 3 times.

8

Stretches for Relief of Heart and Lung Health Issues

When you practice a series of stretching exercises for the upper body, you gently stretch every muscle that affects the expansion of the lungs and the capacity and strength of the heart. These exercises relax tense chest muscles and improve their suppleness and flexibility. They also promote better circulation and oxygenation to tense and contracted areas of the upper body. As a result, general metabolism of this area is improved along with breathing and cardiovascular function.

Deep, slow abdominal breathing is essential for women to boost energy and vitality. It expands your lungs and allows you to bring adequate oxygen, the fuel for metabolic activity, to all the tissues of your body. Rapid, shallow breathing decreases your oxygen supply and keeps you tired and devitalized. Deep breathing helps to stabilize mood and reduce both depression and anxiety, so it is very important for emotional wellbeing.

Exercise 1: Deep Breathing

This exercise helps to relax the entire body and strengthens the muscles in the chest and abdomen.

Lie flat on your back with your knees pulled up. Keep your feet slightly apart. Try to breathe in and out through your nose.

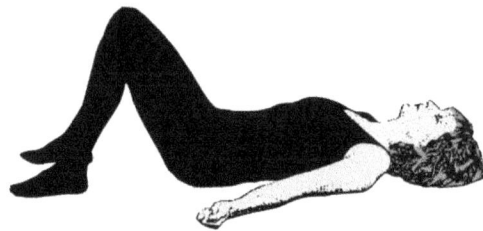

Inhale deeply. As you breathe in, allow your stomach to relax so that the air flows into your abdomen. Your stomach should balloon out as you breathe in.

Visualize your lungs filling up with air so that your chest swells out. Imagine that the air you breathe is filling your body with energy

Exhale deeply. As you breathe out, let your stomach and chest collapse. Imagine the air being pushed out, first from your abdomen and then from your lungs.

Exercise 2

This exercise improves circulation to the upper half of the body and energizes and stimulates it. It also loosens and stretches tense muscles in the upper body, especially the shoulders and back, and expands the lungs.

Stand easily. Arms should be at your sides; feet are hip distance apart.

Bring your arms back slowly and gracefully until you can clasp them behind your back.

Exhale, then straighten your clasped hands and arms as far as you can without discomfort. Remember to stand upright; body should not bend forward. Breathe deeply into chest. Breathe deeply into chest.

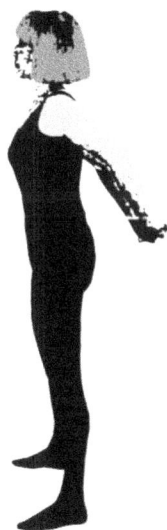

As you hold your breath, bend forward at the waist, bringing your clasped hands and arms up over your back. Relax your neck muscles and keep your knees straight. Hold for a few seconds.

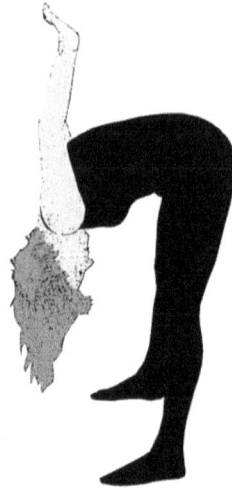

Exhale as you return to the upright position. Unclasp your hands and allow your arms to rest easily at your sides. Repeat sequence 3 times.

9

Stretches for Relief of Anxiety, Panic
Attacks & Stress

Stretches provide effective relief of anxiety and stress. Always perform them slowly and carefully and accompany the stretches with deep, relaxed breathing. Stretches quiet your mood and promote a deep sense of peace and calm. Unlike fast-paced aerobic exercise, stretches actually slow down your pulse, heart rate, and breathing. This benefits many women with anxiety and tension related to life stress. Stretches provides an oasis of calm in which you can put aside your stress and focus on doing the exercises slowly and on breathing calmly and deeply.

Stretch 1

This exercise is excellent for calming anxiety and stress due to emotional causes, and it will also relieve anxiety and irritability due to PMS and menopause. For women with food addiction episodes or coexisting mitral valve prolapse, it will lessen anxiety. This exercise gently stretches the lower back and is one of the most effective exercises for relieving menstrual cramps.

> Sit on your heels. Bring your forehead to the floor, stretching the spine as far over your head as possible. Close your eyes. Hold for as long as comfortable.

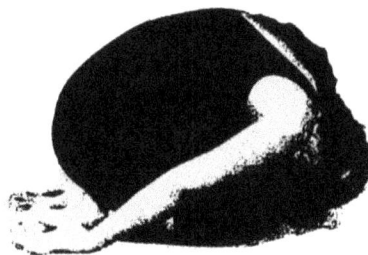

Stretch 2

This exercise relieves anxiety and stress due to emotional causes, PMS, or menopause. It helps quiet anxiety in women with coexisting food addiction episodes or mitral valve prolapse. It relieves menstrual cramps and low back pain. It also reduces eye tension and swelling in the face.

Lie on your back with a rolled towel placed under your knees. Your arms should be at your sides, palms up.

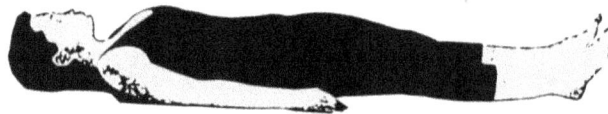

Close your eyes and relax your whole body. Inhale slowly, breathing from the diaphragm. As you inhale, visualize the energy in the air around you being drawn in through your entire body. Imagine that your body is porous and open like a sponge, so it can draw in this energy to revitalize every cell of your body.

Exhale slowly and deeply, allowing every ounce of tension to drain from your body.

Stretch 3

This exercise massages the neck and spine and flexes the vertebral column. It will invigorate and energize you, helping balance your body and mind and reduce fatigue. It also promotes good circulation and relieves low back tension. To enhance the benefits of the exercise, lie flat on your back for a few minutes after doing it.

Lie on your back. Bend and raise your knees to your chest, clasping them with your hands. Hands should be interlocked below knees.

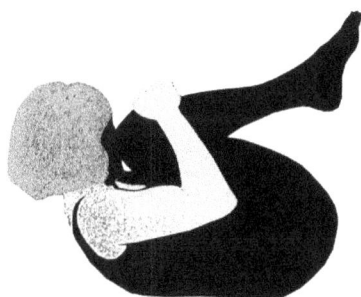

Raise your head toward your knees and gently rock back and forth on your curved spine. Note the roundness of your back and shoulders. Keep the chin tucked in as you roll back. Avoid rolling back too far on your neck.

Rock back and forth 5 to 10 times.

Stretch 4

This pose reduces anxiety and nervous tension and will help eliminate tension headaches and insomnia. It improves flexibility of the spine, reducing stiffness and back pain.

Lie on your back with your legs bent and your feet together. Place your hands on the sides of both ankles to keep your legs together.

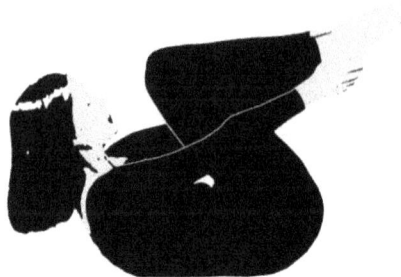

As you inhale, raise your legs up over your head. To make sure that the posture is comfortable, adjust the angle of your legs, bending your knees to apply pressure between the shoulder blades.

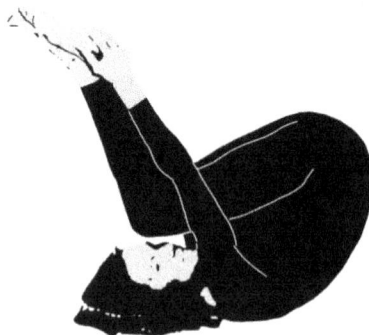

Hold this posture for one minute, breathing slowly and deeply. Return to the original position, lying flat on your back with your eyes closed. Relax in this position for several minutes

Stretch 5

This exercise calms anxiety and nervousness. It strengthens the back and abdominal muscles and improves blood circulation and oxygenation to the pelvis.

Lie down and press the small of your back into the floor. This permits you to use your abdominal muscles without straining your lower back.

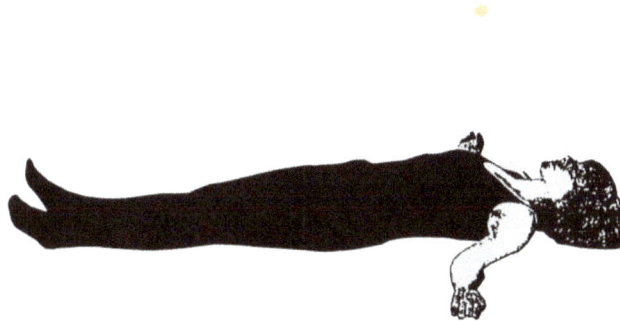

Keep your back flat on the floor and let the rest of your body remain relaxed.

Raise your right leg slowly while breathing in. Move your leg very slowly; imagine your leg being pulled up smoothly by a spring. Do not move your leg in a jerking manner. Hold for a few breaths.

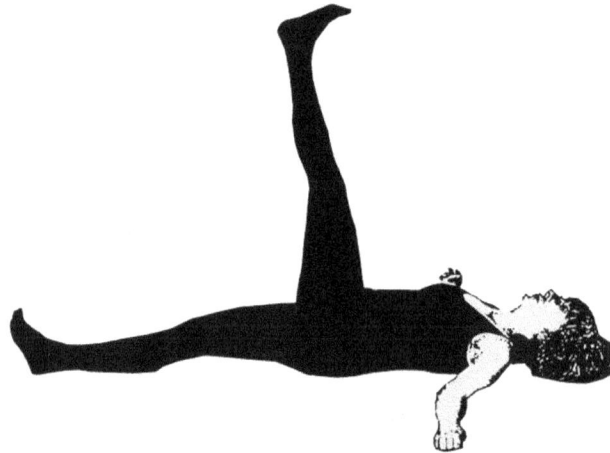

Lower your leg and breathe out. Repeat the same exercise on your left side. Then alternate legs, repeating the exercise 5 to 10 times.

Stretch 6

This exercise reduces anxiety and nervous tension. It also helps to eliminate tension headaches. By stretching the spine, you enhance circulation and improve spinal flexibility.

Lie on your stomach with your chin on the floor and your feet together. Place your palms flat on the floor, underneath your shoulders.

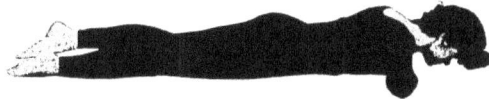

Relax with your head turned to one side and your arms resting gently on the floor.

As you inhale, lift your head up, stretching your neck back. Then, raise your chest, using your arms and back muscles.

As you complete the inhalation, arch your body all the way up, keeping your hips on the ground.

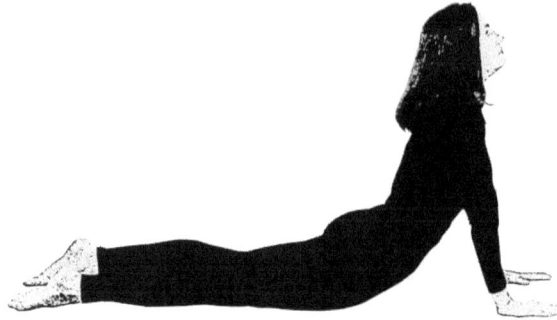

As you hold this position, exhale deeply. Then, breathe deeply and slowly, inhaling and exhaling for 30 seconds.

Lower yourself part way, using your arms for support. Holding the body at this angle, breathe deeply for 30 seconds.

Then let your body come all the way down. Close your eyes and relax for several minutes.

Stretch 7

This exercise helps release overall body tension. It improves circulation and concentration. It strengthens the lower back and abdominal area.

Lie on your stomach with your feet together and your arms lying flat at your sides.

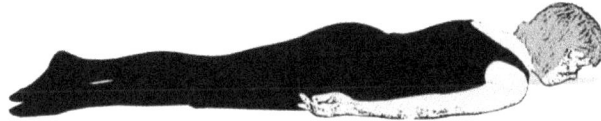

Stretch your arms out straight in front of you on the floor.

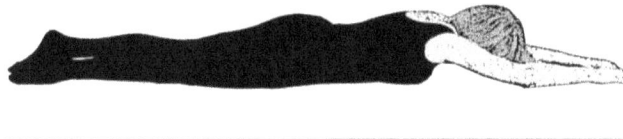

As you inhale, arch your back and lift your arms, head, chest and legs off the floor. Hold the pose as long as you can, up to 30 seconds, breathing deeply and slowly.

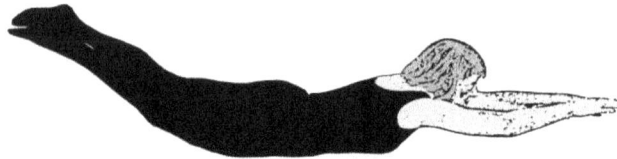

Return to the original resting position with your head turned to the side, and completely relax for 1 to 3 minutes.

Stretch 8

This exercise helps relieve emotional tension and frustration. By helping release emotional upset locked in the muscles, this stretch promotes a sense of relaxation, mental balance, improved energy, and vitality.

Lie on your back with your hands interlaced under your neck. As you inhale, bend and lift your right leg

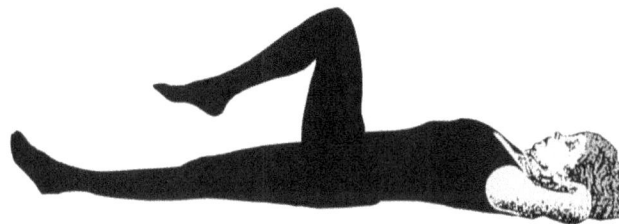

Then exhale and roll on your left side, with your left knee touching the ground. As you do this, release a sigh.

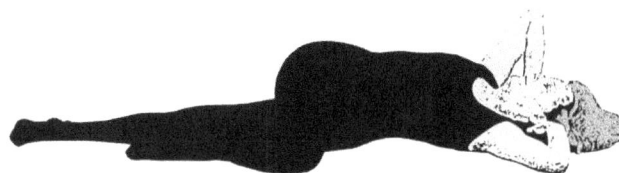

As you inhale, return to your original position. Repeat this 10 times, alternating sides, then relax on your back for 1 minute.

Stretch 9

This exercise helps relieve PMS- and menopause-related anxiety and stress and other premenstrual and menopausal symptoms by energizing the female reproductive tract. It also energizes the liver, intestines, and kidneys, and strengthens the lower back, abdomen, buttocks, and legs.

Lie face down on the floor. Make fists with both your hands and place them under your hips. This prevents compression of the lumbar spine while doing the exercise.

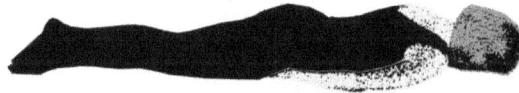

Straighten your body and raise your right leg with a slow upward thrust as high as you can, keeping your hips on your fists. Hold for 5 to 20 seconds if possible.

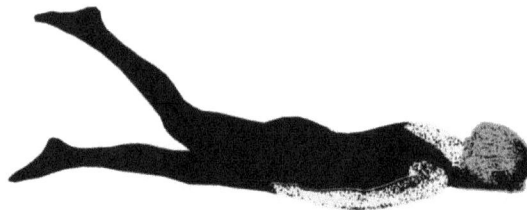

Lower the leg and slowly return to your original position. Repeat with the left leg, then with both legs together. Remember to keep your hips resting on your fists. Repeat 10 times.

Stretch 10

This exercise is one of the most powerful stretches for increasing total body energy and vitality and releasing muscle tension. It strengthens the nervous system, balances the mood, may reduce sugar craving, and helps reduce anxiety and nervous tension. It improves concentration and mental clarity. It also stimulates the thyroid, thymus, liver, kidneys, and female reproductive tract, and improves digestive function.

Lie face down on the floor, arms at your sides.

Slowly bend your legs at the knees and bring your feet up toward your buttocks.

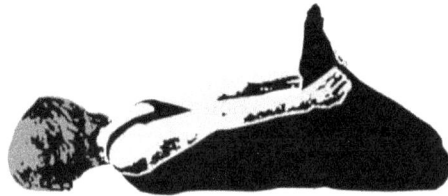

Reach back with your arms and carefully take hold of first one foot and then the other. Flex your feet to make grasping them easier.

Inhale and raise your trunk from the floor as far as possible. Lift your head and elevate your knees off the floor.

Squeeze the buttocks. Imagine your body looking like a gently curved bow. Hold for 10 to 15 seconds.

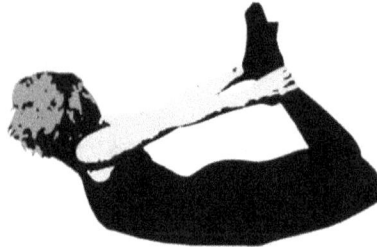

Slowly release the posture. Allow your chin to touch the floor and finally release your feet and return them slowly to the floor. Return to your original position. Repeat 5 times.

Stretch 11

This exercise helps relieve nervous tension and stress, tension headaches, and menstrual problems. It also helps prevent colds and respiratory infections. Use it to relieve allergic and respiratory symptoms.

Lie on your back with your knees bent and the bottoms of your feet flat on the floor.

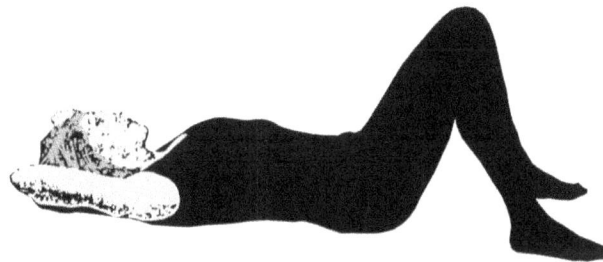

Bring your hands under your neck with the backs of your hands pressing against each other and the knuckles of your smallest fingers pressing into the base of your skull. Spread your index finger and thumb apart on each hand.

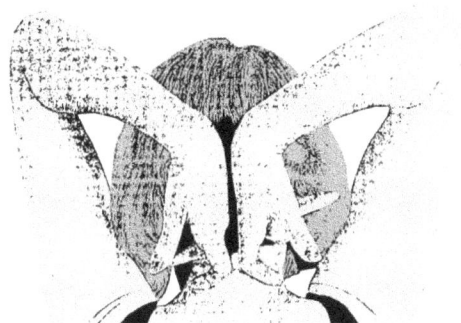

Inhale deeply and arch your hips up. Breathe deeply in this position for up to 1 minute.

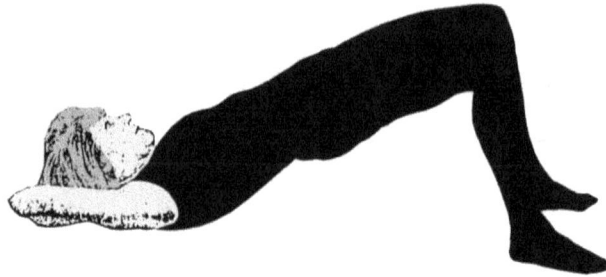

As you exhale, slowly come down and return to your original position. Relax in this position for 1 to 3 minutes.

10

Stretches for Relief of Chronic Fatigue and Depression

I have included in this chapter many different stretches that can improve your level of energy and vitality while you're healing from chronic fatigue or depression. Practiced slowly and gently, these exercises can provide many physiological and emotional benefits for your body. A good stretching routine stretches every muscle in the body, promoting limberness and flexibility in the muscles and joints. At the same time, better circulation and oxygenation to the whole body stimulates metabolism and improves cell function. Improving circulation and nutrient flow to the brain and nervous system promotes healthy brain chemistry. This helps improve your mood, relieve depression, and reduce fatigue.

Best of all, stretching is such an easy and gentle form of exercise that it can be practiced by most people, even women with severe chronic fatigue. Stretching is one of the few forms of physical activity that will not tire out a woman who has low physical reserve and stamina. When practiced on a regular basis, a good stretching routine can be an important part of your self-help program to regain your vigor and vitality.

Stretch 1

This exercise helps relieve fatigue by releasing tension in the shoulder blades. Tension in the shoulders blocks blood flow and oxygenation to the head and neck area, making you feel mentally tired and sluggish.

Stand easily with your legs apart. As you exhale, drop your head and body slowly forward.

Let your fingers hang down as close to the ground as possible. Deep breathe in this position for 30 seconds.

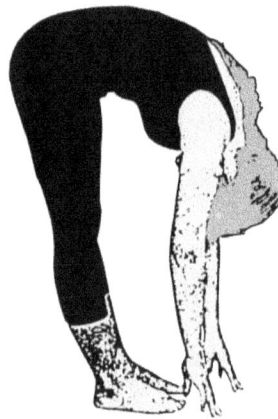

Slowly come up to the standing position. Repeat 3 times.

Stretch 2

This exercise increases circulation to the upper half of the body, energizing and stimulating the body. It also loosens and stretches tense muscles in the upper body, especially the shoulders and back, and expands the lungs.

Stand easily. Arms should be at your sides; feet are hip distance apart.

Bring your arms back slowly and gracefully until you can clasp them behind your back.

Exhale, then straighten your clasped hands and arms as far as you can without discomfort. Remember to stand upright; body should not bend forward. Breathe deeply into chest. Breathe deeply into chest.

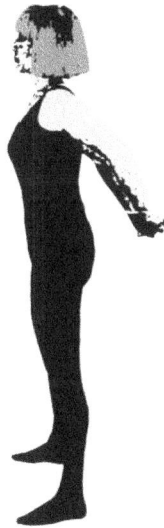

As you hold your breath, bend forward at the waist, bringing your clasped hands and arms up over your back. Relax your neck muscles and keep your knees straight. Hold for a few seconds.

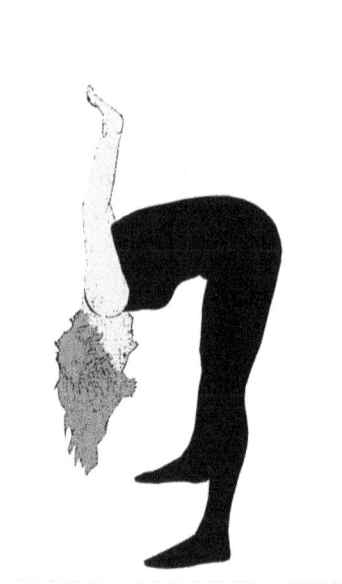

Exhale as you return to the upright position. Unclasp your hands and allow your arms to rest easily at your sides. Repeat sequence 3 times.

Stretch 3

This exercise massages the entire neck, spine, and back muscles, as well as all the acupressure points along the spine. It will help to stimulate a sluggish thyroid by stretching and massaging the neck. This exercise will invigorate and energize you, reducing fatigue.

Lie on your back. Bend and raise your knees to your chest, clasping them with your hands. Hands should be interlocked above knees.

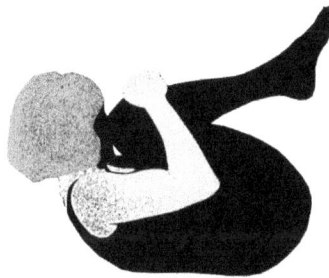

Raise your head toward your knees and gently rock back and forth on your curved spine. Note the roundness of your back and shoulders. Keep the chin tucked in as you roll back. Avoid rolling back too far on your neck. Rock back and forth 5 to 10 times.

Stretch 4

This exercise helps to release overall body tension. It improves circulation and concentration. It helps to strengthen the lower back and abdominal area.

Lie on your stomach with your feet together and your arms lying flat at your sides.

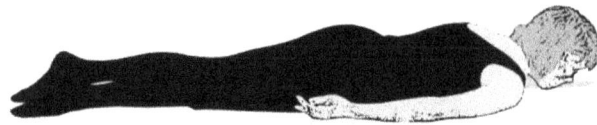

Stretch your arms out straight in front of you on the floor.

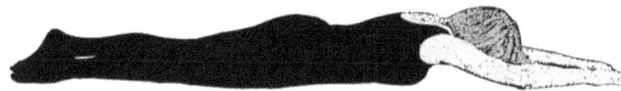

As you inhale, arch your back and lift your arms, head, chest and legs off the floor. Hold the pose as long as you can, up to 30 seconds, breathing deeply and slowly.

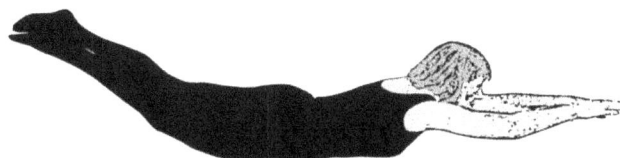

Return to the original resting position with your head turned to the side, and completely relax for 1 to 3 minutes

Stretch 5

This exercise helps relieve PMS fatigue and other premenstrual and menopausal symptoms by energizing the female reproductive tract. It also energizes the liver, intestines, and kidneys. It strengthens the lower back, abdomen, buttocks, and legs.

Lie face down on the floor. Make fists with both your hands and place them under your hips. This prevents compression of the lumbar spine while doing the exercise.

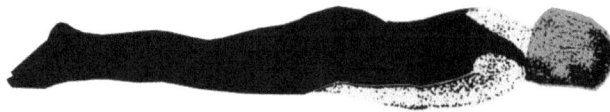

Straighten your body and raise your right leg with an upward thrust as high as you can, keeping your hips on your fists. Hold for 5 to 20 seconds if possible.

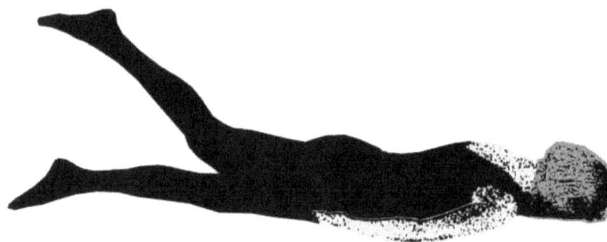

Lower the leg and slowly return to your original position. Repeat on the left side, then with both legs together. Remember to keep your hips resting on your fists. Repeat 10 times.

Stretch 6

This exercise is one of the most powerful stretches for increasing total body energy and vitality and releasing muscle tension. It strengthens the nervous system, improves concentration and mental clarity, and relieves depression. It also stimulates the thyroid, thymus, liver, kidney, and female reproductive tract. It helps to improve digestive function and may reduce sugar craving.

Lie face down on the floor, arms at your sides.

Slowly bend your legs at the knees and bring your feet up toward your buttocks.

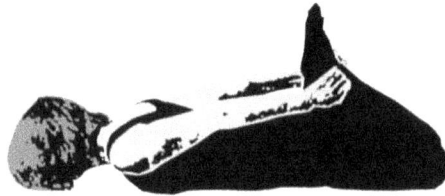

Reach back with your arms and carefully take hold of first one foot and then the other. Flex your feet to make grasping them easier.

Inhale and raise your trunk from the floor as far as possible. Lift your head and elevate your knees off the floor.

Squeeze the buttocks. Imagine your body looking like a gently curved bow. Hold for 10 to 15 seconds.

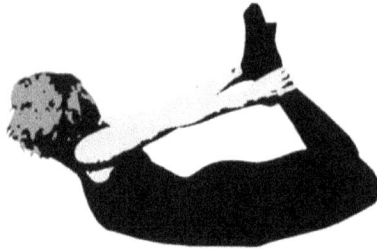

Slowly release the posture. Allow your chin to touch the floor and finally release your feet and return them slowly to the floor. Return to your original position. Repeat 5 times.

Stretch 7

This exercise improves your resistance to infections. Use it to help prevent colds and respiratory infections, to reduce the duration of a cold, or to relieve allergic and respiratory symptoms.

Lie on your back with your knees bent and the bottoms of your feet flat on the floor.

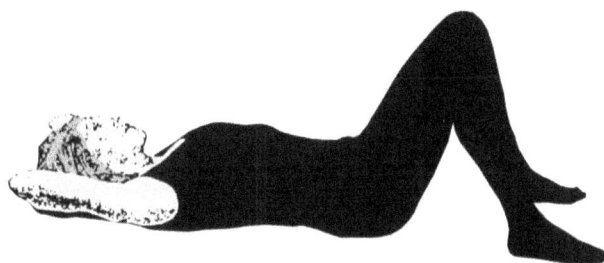

Bring your hands under your neck with the backs of your hands pressing against each other and the knuckles of your smallest fingers pressing into the base of your skull. Spread your index finger and thumb apart on each hand.

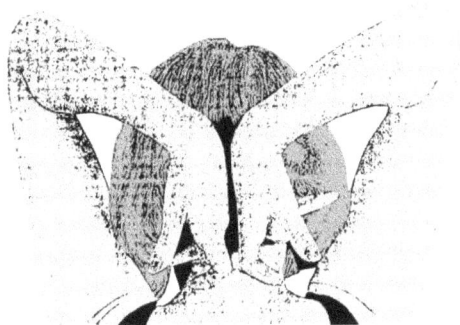

Inhale deeply and arch your hips up. Breathe deeply in this position for up to 1 minute.

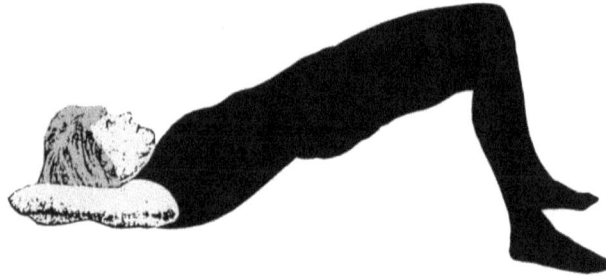

As you exhale, slowly come down and return to your original position. Relax in this position for 1 to 3 minutes.

Stretch 8

This exercise helps increase resistance to infections, particularly colds and flu, as well as decrease fatigue. It also helps clear tension around the shoulder blades.

Sit on your heels, placing the instep of one foot into the arch of the other.

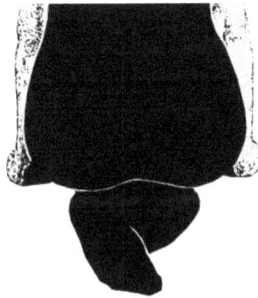

Lower your head slowly forward to the ground, bringing your arms behind your back and interlocking your fingers. Be sure to have your palms facing each other.

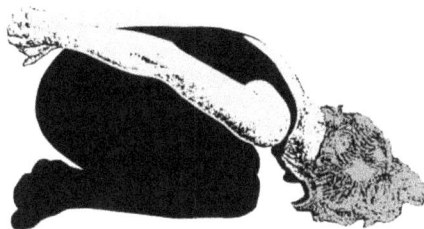

As you inhale, raise your arms straight up, keeping your hands clasped together.

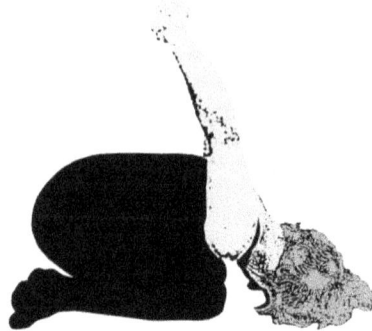

Hold this position for up to 1 minute, breathing deeply.

As you exhale, slowly unclasp your hands and let your arms relax on the floor, palms up.

Relax in this position for 1 to 3 minutes.

Stretch 9

This exercise helps relieve emotional tension and frustration. By helping release emotional upset locked in the muscles, side rolls promote a sense of relaxation, mental balance, and improved energy and vitality.

Lie on your back with your hands interlaced under your neck. As you inhale, bend and lift your right leg.

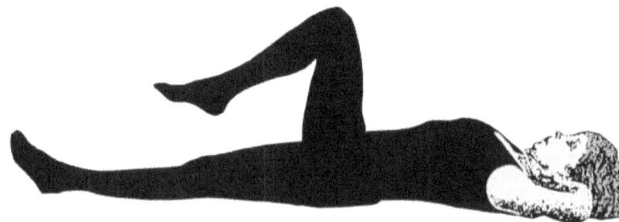

Then exhale and roll on your left side, with your left knee touching the ground. As you do this, release a sigh.

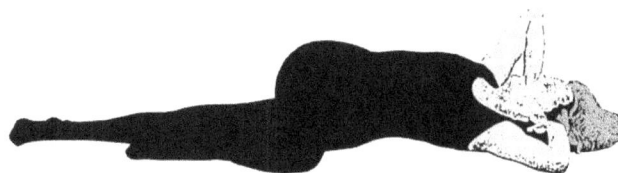

As you inhale, return to your original position. Repeat this 10 times, alternating sides, then relax on your back for 1 minute.

About Susan M. Lark, M.D.

Dr. Susan Lark is one of the foremost authorities in the fields of women's health care and alternative medicine. Dr. Lark has successfully treated many thousands of women emphasizing holistic health and complementary medicine in her clinical practice. Her mission is to provide women with unique, safe and effective alternative therapies to greatly enhance their health and well-being.

A graduate of Northwestern University Feinberg School of Medicine, she has served on the clinical faculty of Stanford University Medical School, and taught in their Division of Family and Community Medicine.

Dr. Lark is a distinguished clinician, author, lecturer and innovative product developer. Through her extensive clinical experience, she has been an innovator in the use of self-care treatments such as diet, nutrition, exercise and stress management techniques in the field of women's health, and has lectured extensively throughout the United States on topics in preventive medicine. She is the author of many best-selling books on women's health. Her signature line of nutritional supplements and skin care products are available through healthydirections.com

One of the most widely referenced physicians on the Internet, Dr. Lark has appeared on numerous radio and television shows, and has been featured in magazines and newspapers including: Real Simple, Reader's Digest, McCall's, Better Homes & Gardens, New Woman, Mademoiselle, Harper's Bazaar, Redbook, Family Circle, Seventeen, Shape, Great Life, The New York Times, The Chicago Tribune, and The San Francisco Chronicle.

She has also served as a consultant to major corporations, including the Kellogg Company and Weider Nutrition International, and was spokesperson for The Gillette Company Women's Cancer Connection.

Dr. Lark can be contacted at (650) 561-9978 to make an appointment for a consultation.

We would enjoy hearing from you! Please share your success stories, requests for new topics and comments with us. Our team at Womens Wellness Publishing may be contacted at yourstory@wwpublishing.com. We invite you to visit our website for Dr. Lark's newest books at womenswellnesspublishing.com.

Dr. Susan's Solutions
Health Library For Women

Women's Health Issues

Dr. Susan's Solutions: Heal Endometriosis

Dr. Susan's Solutions: Healthy Heart and Blood Pressure

Dr. Susan's Solutions: Healthy Menopause

Dr. Susan's Solutions: The Anemia Cure

Dr. Susan's Solutions: The Bladder Infection Cure

Dr. Susan's Solutions: The Candida-Yeast Infection Cure

Dr. Susan's Solutions: The Chronic Fatigue Cure

Dr. Susan's Solutions: The Cold and Flu Cure

Dr. Susan's Solutions: The Fibroid Tumor Cure

Dr. Susan's Solutions: The Irregular Menstruation Cure

Dr. Susan's Solutions: The Menstrual Cramp Cure

Dr. Susan's Solutions: The PMS Cure

Emotional and Spiritual Balance

Breathing Meditations for Healing, Peace and Joy

Dr. Susan's Solutions: The Anxiety and Stress Cure

Women's Hormones

DHEA: The Fountain of Youth Hormone

Healthy, Natural Estrogens for Menopause

Pregnenolone: Your #1 Sex Hormone

Progesterone: The Superstar of Hormone Balance

Testosterone: The Hormone for Strong Bones, Sex Drive and Healthy Menopause

Diet and Nutrition

Dr. Susan Lark's Healing Herbs for Women

Dr. Susan Lark's Complete Guide to Detoxification

Enzymes: The Missing Link to Health

Healthy Diet and Nutrition for Women: The Complete Guide

Renew Yourself Through Juice Fasting and Detoxification Diets

Energy Therapies and Anti-Aging

Acupressure for Women: Relieve Symptoms of Dozens of Health Issues Through Pressure Points

Exercise and Flexibility

Stretching and Flexibility for Women

Stretching Programs for Women's Health Issues

About Womens Wellness Publishing

"Bringing Radiant Health and Wellness to Women"

Womens Wellness Publishing was founded to make a positive difference in the lives of women and their families. We are the premier publisher of print and eBooks focused on women's health and wellness. We are committed to publishing the finest quality and most comprehensive line of books that covers every area that a woman needs to create vibrant health and a joyful, fulfilling life.

Our books are written and created by the top health and wellness experts who share with you, our readers, their wisdom and extensive experience successfully treating many thousands of patients.

We encourage you to browse through our online bookstore; new books are frequently being added at womenswellnesspublishing.com. Also visit our Lifestyle Center and Customer Bonus Center for more exciting and helpful health and wellness information and resources.

Follow us on Facebook for the latest health tips, recipes, and all natural solutions to many women's health issues (facebook.com/wwpublishing).

About Our Associate Program

We invite you to become part of the Womens Wellness Publishing Community through our Associate Program. You will have the opportunity to earn generous commissions on sales that you create through your blog, social network, support groups, community groups, school & alumni groups, friends, family or other networks.

To join our program, go to our website and click "Become an Associate" (womenswellnesspublishing.com). We support your sales and marketing efforts by offering you and your customers:

- Free support materials with updates on all of our new book releases, promotions, and bonuses for you and your customers
- Free audio downloads, booklets, and guides
- Special discounts and sales promotions

www.ingramcontent.com/pod-product-compliance
Lightning Source LLC
Chambersburg PA
CBHW081419270326
41931CB00015B/3334